CARCINOSIN

THE
CARCINOSIN
DRUG PICTURE

by

Dr. D.M. Foubister, M.B., Ch.B., D.C.H., F.F.Hom. (London)
Visiting Physician, Royal London Homoeopathic Hospital;
Formerly Dean of the Faculty of Homoeopathic Education, London.

and

J. Hui Bon Hoa, M.D., D.F.Hom.

B. JAIN PUBLISHERS (P) LTD.

Price: Rs. 25. 00

Ist Edition : 1995
Reprint Edition : 1996, 1997, 1998, 1999, 2001, 2003

Published by:
B. Jain Publishers (P) Ltd.
1921, Street No. 10th Chuna Mandi,
Paharganj, New Delhi-110055 (INDIA)

Printed in India by:
Unisons Techno Financial Consultants (P) Ltd.
522, FIE, Patpar Ganj, Delhi- 110 092.

ISBN : 81-7021-674-5

BOOK CODE : BF-2242

Foreword

I have great pleasure in placing this booklet in the hands of the homoeopathic profession. Dr. D. M. Foubister is a famous homoeopathic physician of whom I have the honour to have been a student. He has made very valuable observations and advances in the homoeopathic treatment of children and some of the essence of his experience is presented herewith. Carcinosin is a remarkable remedy and to Dr. Foubister goes the credit of exploring and exposing its great possibilities. This paper was originally published in the British Homoeopathic Journal and I am deeply grateful both to the editor Dr. L. R. Twentyman and to the author for their kind permission for reprinting this.

P. Sankaran

PREFACE

Various preparations of *Carcinosin* have long been used in homoeopathic practice mainly in cases with a background of a family history of cancer not responding to ordinary constitutional prescribing. The usefulness of *Carcinosin* today may be attributed to the greater amount of radiation to which mankind is exposed or it may be that it can now be prescribed on accurate indications, and was in the past often missed.

All *Carcinosins* have a common action. It may be that the site of the tumour from which a preparation was made can be a guide to the choice, but so far there are no clear differentiating symptoms. It is to be hoped that the unusual approach to discovery of the indications for *Carcinosin* will not put any one off from a clinical trial.

This paper was written some time back but is fully up-to-date. Since then no new indications have emerged, but the ones given below have been further confirmed.

London, January 1967.   **D. M. FOUBISTER**

THE CARCINOSIN DRUG PICTURE

According to homoeopathic philosophy, organic disease is an ultimate, the result of preceding changes in the vitality of the patient which are manifested by functional changes and subjective symptoms. It is generally accepted that organic disease may be foreshadowed by functional changes.[1] It is these symptoms of disordered vitality which have to be matched in selecting a constitutional remedy with the object of correcting the underlying disharmony.

There is perhaps a tendency to regard nosodes representing the ultimates in disease as being comparatively superficial in their action. Yet the well-proved nosodes such as *Tuberculinum* and *Medorrhinum* are undoubtedly among the most deeply acting and valuable medicines in the materia medica. *It may be that nosodes carry in them in their potentized state something of the nature of the preceding deranged vitality.* After six years' study of *Carcinosin* that is my impression and its profound action may possibly be explained in this way. Kent believed cancer to be the result of suppressed psora and it is of interest to note that in some cases responding to *Carcinosin*, indications for *Psorinum* and other anti-psorics not previously evident came to light. In a few cases the symptom of *Psorinum* "feels specially well before an attack" was uncovered only after previous benefit from *Carcinosin*.

My interest in *Carcinosin* was aroused by a chance experience : that of having in the out-patient department simultaneously two children born of mothers who were, during the pregnancy, suffering from cancer of the breast.[2] These children presented a remarkably similar appearance, having blue sclerotics, a café au lait* complexion and numerous moles. Both children suffered from insomnia. I had previously been given a therapeutic hint that where there was a family history of cancer, *Carcinosin* sometimes cured insomnia, and had used it occasionally in insomnia with success.

I wondered if one could regard these children, having been nourished by cancerous blood, as exhibiting these characteristics on account of the mother's condition. In other word was this a sort of proving of *Carcinosin*, or was it a coincidence?

It would take considerable time to collect a number of such cases and the immediate course open was to study the antecedents of children with that appearance to find out whether this appearance was associated with a strong family history of cancer or not. In the out-patient department we began by checking the family history and giving *Carcinosin* to children with that appearance. During the first few years detailed notes were taken by one of my clinical assistants of 200 cases in which we had tested the remedy with or without success. Gradually the picture of *Carcinosin* emerged. It did receive a small proving,[3] and I proved it myself in the 200th potency.

It is generally accepted that we can utilize the symptoms derived from clinical experience of the therapeutic effects of a remedy and that the drug picture

---

* Coffee with milk

which is the real basis of prescribing is built up from provings plus clinical experience.

It has been noted that only a small proportion of provers are sufficiently sensitive to any substance to bring out anything like its full effects, those presumably having an idiosyncrasy to the drug being tested.[4] In studying the therapeutic effects of a homoeopathic remedy one cannot escape the conclusion that anyone benefiting from a drug in high potency must also have been sensitive to it. A more careful study of therapeutic effects would in my view enrich the materia medica. Disease in fact tends to increase sensitivity to the appropriate remedy even in the physiological use of drugs.[5]

It soon became apparent that children of what we came to regard as the "Carcinosin appearance" did not show the kind of family history we had almost expected to find. In many instances there was a strong family history of cancer, but in others there was a strong family history of tuberculosis, of diabetes and pernicious anaemia, or a combination of all these more strongly represented than in the average family; only occasionally there was no such history. It would, of course, require a great deal of research to prove this.

Gradually we gained the impression that in addition to the "Carcinosin appearance" and a tendency to insomnia even in young children there was a tendency to have an inflammatory illness, usually a whooping cough or pneumonia, very early in life, and therefore almost severely. For instance, whooping cough at five months fits into the Carcinosin picture. If, for the sake of argument, we accept McDonagh's concept that there are two basic diseases, inflammation and tumour formation, also the teaching of Rudolf Steiner, then it might not be too far fetched to regard this tendency to inflammation as a reaction against inherited tendencies. A child who had the longest list of severe inflammatory diseases I have ever seen had indications for *Carcinosin,* and its administration was followed by a remarkable improvement. We gained the impression that after administration of *Carcinosin,* there was considerable likelihood of an inflammatory reaction very difficult to prove also without considerable research. in the children's ward Sister Sayer observed that children receiving *Carcinosin* often had a rise of temperature on the tenth day, and this has been often confirmed.

Alimentary upsets of one kind or another, say a tendency to diarrhoea or constipation or acidosis in childhood, seemed to come into the picture, but this is not certain; it is so common in childhood. In the provings Dr. Templeton noted the constancy with which *Carcinosin* produced constipation.

In the children's ward we observe the position in which a child sleeps, and in the out-patient department I have for years asked all mothers about this symptom, as it is an unequivocal one. There is a tendency for many infants to sleep in the knee-elbow position up to the last quarter of the first year, then it often disappears. The knee-elbow position is noted in *Kent's Repertory* only under *Medorrhinum,* but our enquiry has revealed that a number of drugs have it. *Carcinosin* has this symptom (also a tendency to sleep on the back, hands above head). Other drugs having the knee-elbow position, which is obviously more valuable as a symptom in older children, are *Tuberculinum, Phosphorus, Sepia, Lycopodium* and *Calc. phos.*

More work is required to elucidate the full picture

of mentals and generals of *Carcinosin*, but clinical studies gradually revealed that *Carcinosin* is related to some of the most commonly indicated and deeply acting medicines in the materia medica and the action of *Carcinosin* is deep and long lasting.

The majority of the children in out-patient had been receiving treatment, and it became apparent that many children who were candidates for *Carcinosin* in other respects had already been helped by one or more of a group of remedies, the most constant of which are *Tuberculinum, Medorrhinum, Nat. mur.* and *Sepia.* Others were *Alumina, Ars. alb., Ars. iod., Pulsatilla, Staphisagria, Phos., Calc. phos., Lueticum, Lycopodium, Sulphur, Psorinum, Dysentery co.* and *Opium.* Others may be added as experience grows.

In any patient not responding to one of these remedies, though accurately chosen, it is worthwhile to see whether *Carcinosin* may fit the case. Also, when two or more of the related remedies are partially indicated but no one adequately covers the case, *Carcinosin* should be considered. These indications for *Carcinosin* have been abundantly confirmed.

Say, you have a child with the obstinacy and love of travel of *Tub. bov.* combined with amelioration by the sea and other symptoms of *Medorrhinum,* a fairly common combination in my experience. *Carcinosin* will often cover the case. I have not hesitated to prescribe *Carcinosin* at the beginning of treatment if clearly indicated, with excellent results.

The provings elicited very little except dullness of mind, thinking difficult, disinterested, aversion to conversation and one can link up *Carcinosin* with *Medorrhinum* in the treatment of backward or mentally defective children. Clarke noted that *Carcinosin* was useful in mental cases with a tendency to suicide and family history of cancer.

In my experience with *Carcinosin*, it is useful in mental cases with a background of fright, prolonged fear, or unhappiness. Fear can come into the picture a great deal, and anticipation. This is an important aspect of *Carcinosin*.

Among the specific mental symptoms it covers is **Fastidiousness**. Think of its related remedy, *Arsenicum*. It can be added to the tidy remedies *Ars., Nux, Anacardium, Graphites*. It can have the opposite being related to *Sulphur*.

It has the obstinacy of *Tub. bov.* and the enjoyment watching a thunderstorm of *Sepia*. It has the marked sense of rhythm, the love of dancing of *Sepia*. It has the sensitivity to music of *Sepia,* and the sympathy others of *Phos.* etc., also incidentally a feature of *Sepia*.

It has in children the sensitivity to reprimand of *Medorrhinum* and other, if not all, sycotics.

GENERALS : Among physical generals *Carcinosin* has either a craving or an aversion to one or more of the following:

Salt, Milk, Eggs, Fat meat, Fruit

and there may be a craving now and an aversion at another time in the same patient not an uncommon finding in childhood.

It can be added, therefore, to the small list of remedies having a desire for meat fat.

. *Carcinosin* has alternation of symptoms like *Lac caninum, Sepia* etc.

Regarding environment influences, *Carcinosin* is better or worse from sea air.

This is a very definite symptom linking it up with *Medorrhinum, Nat. mur.,* and *Sepia,* also *Tuberculinum* which sometimes is worse at the seaside.

Discounting the benefit of a rest for the tired housewife, the exhilaration of the child going to the coast for its annual holiday, and the influence of fresh air on the town dweller, sea air does greatly ameliorate some patients and their asthma or peptic ulcer pain disappears regularly by the seaside, or it may have the opposite effect.

We should, however, be careful not to accept as absolutely definite the symptoms recorded in *Kent's Repertory* under "Air, Sea". *Medorrhinum* almost invariably is ameliorated by the sea but very rarely it is worse by the sea. *Nat. mur.* is about 50-50. It is benefited by sea air just as often as it is aggravated.

Carcinosin is worse or better at the seaside and quite often is worse at the East Coast and better on the South Coast or vice versa.

A word about the various preparations of *Carcinosin.* The original *Carcinosin,* obtainable at Nelson's and Keene & Ashwell, is the one which was proved and the one which we have used mainly. Its source is unknown, but it is believed to be from *carcinoma* of breast. Recently two new series of preparations have been made by Nelson's to whom we have supplied specimens from the homoeopathic hospital, and Gould & Son who have potentized a number of specimens of cancer obtained from another source.

In general it may be said that the recently introduced preparations are much more active, and there is a very definite place for the newer ones. Of these I have had most experience with Nelson's *Carcinosin adenostom,* and it is a very powerful nosode. Gould's preparations are also extremely active and valuable.

Another point in the prescription of *Carcinosin* as a constitutional remedy is that it is probably unsafe to give it to patients suspected of cancer. It has been frequently used in the treatment of cancer. In one article in an old *Homoeopathic Recorder* it is claimed to ease the pain of cancer of the breast. It is not easy to find a single case of cancer treated by *Carcinosin* alone, and it seems to be of very doubtful value in the treatment of the disease. In fact, *it almost seems that the further away you get from actual cancer, as in childhood, the more useful Carcinosin is a constitutional remedy.*

SUMMARY

HEREDITARY BACKGROUND: Various preparations of *Carcinosin* have long been used in homoeopathic practice, mainly on the indication of a strong family history of cancer. Recent clinical experience suggests that they may be useful as constitutional remedies for patients having a strong family history of cancer, diabetes, tuberculosis, or a mixture of these diseases, more strongly represented than in an "average" family.

RELATED REMEDIES: *The Tuberculins, Medorrhinum, Syphilinum, Sepia, Natrum muriaticum, Calcarea phosphorica, Dys. co., Lycopodium, Phosphorus, Psorinum, Arsenicum album, Arsenicum iodatum,Pulsatilla, Sulphur, Opium, Alumina* and *Staphysagria.*

(a) There may be partial indications for two or more of these remedies without complete coverage by any single one, such as the desire for travel of

Tuberculinum or *Calcarea phosphorica;* the fastidiousness of *Arsenicum album;* and the dislike of consolation of *Natrum muriaticum* or *Sepia.* Many combinations may be found.

(b) One of these remedies may apparently be clearly indicated, e.g. *Sepia* and little effect is produced, or the effect may be short-lived. Sometimes a series of those remedies may have been given without really satisfactory results.

APPETITE : There may be a craving for, or aversion to salt, milk, eggs, fat, fruit (N.B.—It can be added to the list of remedies having a craving for fat).

ENVIRONMENT: A definite symptom which has emerged is "influenced by sea air". The patient may be better or worse at the seaside, or may be better at the East Coast and worse at the South Coast and vice versa, as a *Carcinosin* indication.

POSITION IN SLEEP IN CHILDREN : The knee-elbow position is covered by *Medorrhinum, Carcinosinum, Calcarea phosphorica, Phosphorus, Sepia, Lycopodium* and probably others. Normally this position is adopted in the first nine or twelve months of life, then it is less often found and is therefore of more value when found in older children.

PERSONAL HISTORY : There is often tendency to insomnia even in childhood. Whooping cough or pneumonia frequently occur early in life and therefore tend to be severe.

APPEARANCE OF THE PATIENT : Interest was aroused by the similarity between two children born of mothers who while pregnant were suffering from cancer of the breast and subsequently died from it. These children had a brownish, *café au lait* complexion, numerous moles and blue sclerotics. Both suffered from insomnia (the *Carcinosins* are useful remedies for insomnia, when indicated).

SUGGESTIVE OF THE CARCINOSINS AS CONSTITUTIONAL REMEDIES :

One or more of the following:

(a) The family history (and possibly the personal history).

(b) Reaction to sea air.

(c) Appetite.

(d) Knee-elbow position in children.

(e) Related remedies. Either two or more strong partial indications, or, one or more remedies have not achieved what would be expected.

(f) The patient's appearance.

All the *Carcinosins* have a general common action, as outlined above, but it is likely that further experience will demonstrate points of differentiation.

CASE HISTORIES

Case 1: A girl of 10 years was first seen in 1952 with a history of asthma dating from a fright caused by a flying-bomb when she was 18 months old. After orthodox treatment the parents took her to an osteopath and after he too failed, she arrived at Shepherd's Bush Clinic.

PREVIOUS ILLNESS : Pneumonia at 1 year. Whooping cough badly at 9 years, followed by an aggravation of the asthma for 6 months.

FAMILY HISTORY : Diabetes on both sides of the mother's family.

No history of cancer.

MENTALS, GENERALS : Weeps if reprimanded.

Aversion to fat meat and eggs. Also allergic to eggs and intolerant he smell of eggs.

Asthma better at seaside.

APPEARANCE : *Café au lait* complexion. Numerous moles. Blue sclerotics.

Carcinosin was followed by an aggravation and then a sustained improvement in health. During the past five years she has had altogether four doses of *Carcinosin* 200 and one of 1 m. The only other medicine on the card is *Phos.* 6 for some acute condition. She is now discharged, having had eight minor attacks since the beginning of treatment and none for the past year.

Case 2: Another child who had the typical appearance and in this case no family history of any of the related diseases.

She was seen first at the age of 11 about two years ago, having been discharged from a teaching hospital with second stage nephritis following a severe acute attack. The urine had 6 parts albumen per 1,000, a few granular casts, many leucocytes and lower urinary tract epithelial cells. Blood urea 22 mgm per cent. This had persisted for some time and a very gloomy prognosis had been given.

PREVIOUS ILLNESS : Whooping cough, measles, tonsillitis, enuresis—slow in getting dry.

FAMILY HISTORY: Nil.

MENTALS, GENERALS: Typical appearance, *café au lait* complexion, numerous moles, very blue sclerotics.

Desires salt, eggs (vinegar, coffee).

Aversion to milk.

Sleeps well.

Carcinosin 30, 200, 1m was given, and a month later seen by someone else at the hospital who gave *Sepia* 12.

There was a great improvement in general health and the albumen went down fairly rapidly to 1 part per 1,000 and the urine was otherwise normal. Eventually there was just a persistent trace of albumen. Ten months later with this trace of albumen *B coli mutabile* 200 was given, and the next specimen a month later was clear.

That is over a year ago, and there has been no recurrence of albumen.

Case 3: This illustrates the use of *Carcinosin* in a case where an apparently well-selected related remedy, *Nat. mur.,* failed to produce a lasting effect. This man of 50 came to see me about two years ago with the complaint of asthma for eight years.

PREVIOUS ILLNESS : Migraine, which ceased before the asthma developed. Concussion at the age of 21. Tonsils and adenoids removed as a child.

FAMILY HISTORY: Mother, cancer of bowel. Father, peptic ulcer.

MENTALS and GENERALS : Sympathetic to others. Sensitive to music.

Tired in the sun (sensitive to drugs, especially acids).

Aversion to salt.

Better in himself in the evening.

Asthma worse in wet weather; worse at 10 a.m., better cool dry days.

Nat. mur. 30, 200, 1 m was given and followed by a definite improvement but he relapsed within two weeks.

Nat. mur. 200, 1 m, 10 m, was tried with some improvement and another quick relapse. Then *Nat. sulph.* 200 was tried but without any real benefit.

Thinking over the case it seemed to me that *Nat. mur.* would ordinarily have had a much better effect in this case. It did have an excellent effect which vanished after two weeks, and apart from *Nat. sulph.* which also failed, there did not appear to be any other obvious remedy. Taking into consideration the relationship of Nat. mur. to *Carcinosin* and the history of his mother having died of cancer, *probably a stronger heredity indication than any other, Carcinosin* 30 was followed by several months of freedom from asthma and another dose by a further period of several months of freedom up to the present, and great benefit to general health.

Case 4: Another case already reported in the paper of 1954 further illustrates the use of *Carcinosin* when an apparently well-indicated remedy failed, in this case *Sepia.*

A woman of 30 suffered from boils in the ears, alternating from one ear to the other. Chemotherapy helped to clear up the boils but did not stop recurrence. She had no freedom from boils for more than a week or two at a time. The following symptoms were present : Disliked consolation, could not weep even when she lost her mother who died from cancer of the uterus. Nausea and vomiting at the beginning of her periods. Dragging down at M.P. Headache before a thunderstorm. Tired in the morning, better in the evening. Profuse offensive axillary perspiration. *Nat. mur.* and *Gelsemium* have sadness but cannot weep. *Sepia,* however, which contains *Nat. mur.,* seemed to be much more indicated. The patient was given *Sepia* 30, 200, 1m on three consecutive days. She had a week's aggravation, then six weeks' freedom and her menstrual symptoms were relieved. She was then given *Sepia* 200, 1m, 10m, which was followed by three weeks of freedom, after which another relapse. *Carcinosin* 30, 200, 1m was given.

It was followed by a severe aggravation lasting about a week and then had been followed by complete freedom for three years.

Case 5: The next case is that of a girl of 15 years of age who had practically all her life a chronic yellow nasal catarrh and frequent colds. Her condition had been worse since whooping cough at the age of 11 years.

PREVIOUS ILLNESS : Tonsils and adenoids removed. Measles badly. Whooping cough very badly.

All childish illnesses more severe than her five sibs.

FAMILY HISTORY : Mother subsequently died of cancer of oesophagus.

MENTALS, GENERALS : Timid, loves affection, chews nails.

Very fond of dancing.

Terrific reader.

Feels a fright in her stomach.

Starts at noise. Anticipation or chlorine in a swimming bath starts up eczema. Anticipation may cause vomiting.

Carcinosin appearance.

Pulsatilla and *Sepia* were considered, but in view of her appearance and the severe whooping cough and the fact that both *Pulsatilla* and *Sepia* are related to *Carcinosin,* she was given *Carcinosin adenostom* 30, 200, 1 m, the *C. adenostom* being selected because of fright in the stomach and vomiting on anticipation.

There was a violent aggravation after which catarrh and colds vanished for a year.

Case 6: A child of 9 suffered from the age of 5 months from recurrent attacks of fever going up to 104°-105°, not influenced by any orthodox drugs. Investigation in two hospitals had proved negative.

The picture was that of a typical attack of acidosis—the periodic syndrome—including the fect that they never lasted for more than five days, and attacks could come on from excitement. The attacks were followed by a loss of weight, and the parents had no real confidence in homoeopathy but had come out of a sense of duty to clutch at the very last straw. There was nothing outstanding in the personal or family history except that the attacks came on a month after vaccination at 3 months and the father had suffered from similar attacks in childhood which cleared up before puberty.

In this case the best course seemed to be to try to stop the attacks first to gain the parents' confidence and then treat constitutionally.

Belladonna 30 was administered on the symptomatology 3 hourly for the first 24 hours, then 6 hourly for two days.

There were an enormous mass of prescribing symptoms, far too many, and the parents did not seem to understand what was wanted. To cut a long story short, *Belladonna* helped enormously to cut down the severity and length of the attacks and then *Calc. phos.* 30, 200, 1m given with partial success in reducing the number of attacks. Later *Carsinosin adenostom* 200 was given about a year ago and there has only been one slight attack in the past six months. The main indications here were a combination of related remedies including *Calc. phos.* Among her symptoms were : Loves a thunderstorm, likes fruit and fat meat as well as bacon fat. Loves affection. Suffers from anticipation. Dreams of snakes. Sensitive to reprimand. Mentally tense (*Dys. co.*).

Case 7: A boy of 13 years had suffered from asthma from the age of 2, both spasmodic and bronchial attacks.

PREVIOUS ILLNESS : Three attacks of pneumonia at 3 months, 10 months and 18 months of age. Asthma started after the second pneumonia.

FAMILY HISTORY: Nil, except tendency to asthma on father's side. Dissimilar twin brother also had asthma for which he was given *Medorrhinum,* which cured him.

MENTALS AND GENERALS : *Carcinosin* appearance; moles +++

Sensitive to reprimand.

Loves fat meat.

Asthma always better at the seaside.

In this case *Medorrhinum* seemed indicated except for the love of fat meat—an example of two or more partial indications for related remedies.

Carcinosin 200 was given and during the following year he had only two minor attacks.

Case 8: A girl of 9 was brought with the complaint of night terrors for five years. She had a severe fright at 2, when her tonsils and adenoids had been removed.

The mother described the terrors: She screams while still asleep; when wakened she answers correctly and forgets about the episode in the morning. On one occasion she talked of being afraid of someone behind a screen.

PREVIOUS ILLNESS : Nil.

FAMILY HISTORY : Nil.

The child was of the *Phosphorus* type—responsive, affectionate, wanting to please and the kind of night terrors might well have been covered by *Phos.*, but she had other symptoms not covered by *Phos.* which were quite definite.

Loves dancing. Very tidy.

(Sympathetic to animals only).

Phosphorus was given with some definite benefit, later *Opium* to antidote the fright, and eventually *Carcinosin*, and the night terrors disappeared for two years altogether. Then the adenoids grew in again and another operation was done, and back came the terrors which again were abolished by *Carcinosin* 30, 200, 1m.

Case 9: Another case I will just briefly mention. A boy of 14, much underweight, had been severely frightened ever since going to a boarding school at 9. Among his symptoms was fear of people, fear of mirrors, and he "bottled things up". *Staphysagria, Stramonium* and later *Medorrhinum* helped. Eventually *Carcinosin* was given at long intervals and he is now doing his military training and has recently passed the stiff physical tests for a commission.

Case No. 10: Mrs. R. 45. Married. Generalized early osteoarthritis, hands, feet, spine.

PREVIOUS ILLNESS: Recurrent pseudocyesis with enlarged abdomen and milk in breasts.

Tubes ligated on advice of psychiatrist.

Prolonged fear in childhood caused by a sadistic father.

Used to stammer.

Still cannot say certain words including number 8 or letters.

FAMILY HISTORY: Nil.

MENTALS AND GENERALS : Sympathetic to others and loves affection. Sentimental.

Headache in thunderstorm.

Loves dancing. Sensitive to certain people.

Weak ankles.

(Still afraid in dark). Never weeps.

8-6-57 *Carcinosin* 30, 200, 1 m given with remarkable benefit and patient can say "8" now.

28-9-57, *Sepia* 12, also *Ruta.*

Iron in low potency.

Case 11: Egyptian boy of 5 years. Recurrent colds, debility. Tonsils removed at 2 years.

PREVIOUS ILLNESS : No illnesses.

FAMILY HISTORY: *Both parents cancer.*

GENERALS AND MENTALS: *Carcinosin* appearance (many moles). Obstinate. Sensitive to music. Loves travel.

Aversion fat cream +. Aversion salt.

Sensitive to reprimand.

Perspires profusely even in winter, *Carcinosin* 30, 200, 1 m given 4-5-54. Letter, December 6th, 1954, from his father:

"The temperature foreseen by you appeared on the 15th day and lasted 24 hours. He has developed physical endurance and there has been no more snoring or coughing. As a matter of fact, John has not had a single cold until lately and this is most exceptional, particularly in view of the debilitating climate we have to endure here (East Africa)."

Case 12: Finally, a tragic case of cancer in childhood. It is of interest from the view-point of the *Carcinosin* drug picture.

A child of 11 years of age was looking after a baby in a garden, the gate of which opened into a *cul de sac*. The baby managed to slip out through the gate while the girl looking after her was preoccupied, and was killed by a motor car. The girl was so shocked she stopped growing, and eventually developed cancer of the liver from which she died.

THE FAMILY HISTORY was as follows : Father's mother died of pernicious anaemia. Father's brother died of cancer. Mother's mother died of diabetes.

PREVIOUS ILLNESS; Measles only.

MENTALS AND GENERALS : Loves affection. Sympathetic to others. Very tidy. Blue sclerotics. Numerous moles. *Café au lait* complexion.

In conclusion, I wish to thank those who have contributed to this clinical study, especially Dr. James Hamilton, Dr. Andrew Strigner and Dr. L. R. Twentyman.

REFERENCES

(1) Kent, J. T.: Lectures on Homoeopathic Philosophy.

(2) Foubister, D. M.: "Clinical Impressions of Carcinosin", *Brit. Hom. J. 44,* April, 1954.

(3) Templeton, W. L.: *Brit. Hom. J. 44,* April 1954. (4) Goodman and Gilman: *The Pharmacological Basis of Therapeutics* 1955, p. 12, Macmillan & Co.

(5) *Ibid,* pp. 12 and 13.

(6) Templeton, W. L.: *Brit. Hom. J.). 44,* April 1954.

DISCUSSION

THE PRESIDENT, Dr. A. D. MacNeill, expressed the thanks of the meeting to Dr. Foubister for his most interesting paper and said he was interested in .the relationship between *Carcinosin* and other remedies which had been mentioned. He then opened the meeting to discussion.

DR. T. D. Ross said that this paper had given us a great deal of material. The interesting thing was that Dr. Foubister was using *Carcinosin* as a remedy for constitutions to make healthier people, in particular starting in childhood. This, of course, was the best time to treat patients in order to prevent serious disease in the future. The use of *Carcinosin* in actual cancer had not produced such brilliant results. This is as we would expect because in these cases we are dealing with ultimate disease processes. Or are we? In fact some of those developing cancer have quite good heredity and past history. Many, however, have bad health and may be nervous or asthmatic or have a bad heredity. In these

Carcinosin is very valuable and one links it with *Medorrhinum*. He thought the stress on family history was important and should be more universally adopted in history taking. He also thought we ought to try using the newer more potent preparations of *Carcinosin*. Nelson's original *Carcinosin* had come. from America and Dr. Compton Burnett got his from Epps, Thatcher. All these comments linked up with the virus theory of cancer. Are we perhaps using a virus or infecting agent along with antibodies? In our *Carcinosin* maybe pure virus would be better and the method of preparation may be important. Several serums have been prepared for cancer in the past, other than homoeopathic ones.

DR. FOUBISTER said that he wishes to warn us about the new preparations as these were very potent and could cause violent reaction, but in suitable cases worked very well indeed.

DR. AHMAD asked why we used the 30, 200 and 1m potencies in series.

DR. FOUBISTER replied that he thought this probably caused less aggravation than the single dose.

DR. CAMPBELL described a case of pernicious anaemia she had in 1945 and had treated with *Carcinosin* 200, 3 doses weekly together with *Ars. alb.* and *Ferr. phos.* 6x repeated. This patient had been unable to go out or do any work. She was now well and able to undertake quite a lot. She had had no vitamin B12.

DR. RUNCIE said he was interested in the relationship of cancer to an inflammatory state. Is it not helpful to induce an inflammatory condition in order to get a result, as there is a lack of inflammation in cancer? He quoted a case of a lady with ganglia on her wrist, one of which had been cut, but it recurred. She was treated with *Benz. acid* for a long time and the other ganglia disappeared. The one which had been cut remained. He discovered, however, a history of miscarriage and prescribed *Pyrogen*. The ganglion eventually cleared up.

DR. FOUBISTER stated that an inflammatory state also occurs after using *Iscador* in cancer. He had used *Carcinosin* in cases of ganglion.

DR. COOPER said he thought of *Carcinosin* if there was a history of syphilitic heredity and stated that he knew of a certain island which had an epidemic of syphilis in 1870 and there was now much cancer, hypertension and mental illness of depressive type. He wondered if *Carcinosin* and *Lueticum* might be closely related.

To which DR. FOUBISTER replied that he thought this was most likely, and these remedies were probably complementary.

DR. DUTHIE said we were most fortunate in having heard Dr. Foubister as he had given us something that we could not get else where. Burnett had originally introduced eleven *Carcinosins*. He had also found that *Nat. mur,* was a complement to *Carcinosin*. He thought that *Thuja* "woke up" his patients. He had found Dr. Foubister's remarks on modalities most interesting. He also stated that Clarke mentioned that milk should not be given and salt should be eliminated from the diet of patients with cancer, as this seemed to stimulate tissue activity.

DR. STEWART remarked that he thought *Carcinosin* should not be used in actual cases of cancer. This was in keeping with other nosodes. Burnett had found that *Bacillinum* was not much help in established cases of tuberculosis.

He then went on to the enjoyment of all by reciting.

Carcinosins The Ballad of Cars and Sins

Begins with car which makes you think of going away.

So travelling appeals to some of these poor souls.

The car begins with "C" which stands for *café au lait*

Complexion as well as cutaneous moles.

He craves or cannot take at all

Egg, fruit, fat, and also sal.

"C" stands for consolation causing distress

And consummate correctness and fastidiousness.

Carcinosin's last syllable starts with "S"

And sin makes you think of sleeplessness,

"S" stands for the spots on which they rest,

Elbows and knees which you've probably guessed,

"S" stands for sea and sclerotics that are blue.

DR. GORDON ROSS said that he had now a much clearer idea of the *Carcinosin* type. He often used it in a new case in a child in order to prepare the ground for other remedies. He had recently had three cases of bad hearts in children in which he had used this remedy whose mothers were *Nat. mur.* cases.

DR. FOUBISTER said that he had found it valuable in rheumatic fever as many of these children have a *café au lait* appearance. He also thought it was necessary to repeat the remedy weekly in these cases. One might often start with *Carcinosin* and then obtain a clear indication for other remedies. He thought that more than one remedy was usually required in treatment.

DR. T. D. ROSS asked if he had any experience of its use in cases of worms, and DR. FOUBISTER replied that he had used it sometimes but was not sure how it compared with Burnett's Scirrhinum.

DR. E. PATERSON said she thought *Carsinosin* was the end result of all miasms and this was why often *Tub., Medorrhinum* and *Lueticum* were all needed. Regarding Dr. Foubister's remarks that nosodes might be deep or superficial, she thought they were always deep. She also wondered how soon one should repeat the *Carcinosin*. She remembered a case of a baby with a skin which had been greatly irritated by a nosode and she felt this could not be left without some kind of treatment while the aggravation was wearing off.

To this DR. FOUBISTER replied that when he mentioned superficial he meant e.g. using *B. coli mutabile* for clearing up the remains of urinary infection. He thought that *Carcinosin* could be repeated in the same way as other remedies. Sometimes the mental symptoms of *Puls.* or *Staph.* may come out in children after *Carcinosin* and he wondered whether he should prescribe the remedy or wait.

Regarding the skin irritation, he sometimes used hydrocortisone ointment etc. in these cases, because he felt that the emotional upset of itch might well effect the action of the remedy.

DR. GUNN said she was rather afraid of *Carcinosin* but had used it very successfully in repeated dosage 3x for cases of chronic mastitis.

DR. BOYD remarked that much stress had been placed on the appearance of these children, and he for one had not come across very many with the typical *café au lait* colour, moles and blue sclerotics, and he wondered whether perhaps these were not as clear as one gathered from Dr. Foubister's paper. He also queried Dr. Stewart's statement regarding the use of nosodes in acute disease, as he had successfully helped a child with primary tuberculosis with three doses of *Tub. bov.* 12c which had brought down the fever and cleared up the chest.

DR. STEWART replied that he had been quoting Burnett on use of *Bacillinum* in late cases.

DR. FOUBISTER said that the appearance might be fully or only partially in evidence. If it were present, at least in this country it was a very suggestive pointer, but its partial or even complete absence, as in the case of other characteristic symptoms, should not deter one from prescribing *Carcinosin* providing it was indicated on other grounds such as family history, failure of related remedies though apparently well indicated, or indications for two or more of the related —remedies without complete coverage by one.

The meeting finished with a vote of thanks to Dr. Foubister for his most interesting paper.

Postscript 1967

The indications for *Carcinosin* outlined above have been verified and further information has been obtained. The late Dr. Douglas Ross considered *Carcinosin* to be essentially a sycotic remedy, which is understandable from its origin, although it covers all miasms. Dr. Paschero and Dr. Shapiro independently found that *Carcinosin* can be added to the list of homoeopathic medicines most generally indicated for adverse after-effects of vaccination. Dr. Paschero also had the opportunity to administer *Carcinosin* preoperatively to patients undergoing plastic surgery, and found that the incidence of keloid scars was greatly reduced.

Dr. Hui Bon Hoa who has had extensive experience with *Carcinosin* stressed its high value to patients unduly disturbed by anticipation, and here again it can be added to the list of homoeopathic medicines suitable for "complaints from anticipation".

In slow recovery from any acute illness, miasmatic influences require consideration. *Carcinosin* has been found useful in this sphere in general, when indicated, but especially in cases of whooping cough not responding to apparently indicated remedies. Glandular fever may run a prolonged course, and it may not be easy to make accurate homoeopathic prescriptions because the protean nature of the pathology makes it difficult or impossible to distinguish between pathological and reactive symptoms. Some years ago a young woman presented herself for treatment of sub-acute glandular fever. She was typically *Carcinosin* in her constitutional make-up, and the superficial resemblance between groups of enlarged lymph glands in this disease and malignancy seemed to be an additional indication. Administration of *Carcinosin* 200, was followed by a lasting improvement. Ten consecutive cases were subsequently treated in the sub-acute stage with *Carcinosin,* and nine cases showed considerable improvement.

Another aspect of *Carcinosin* which was noted during the clinical proving was that when indicated, amelioration or cure might be obtained, or if a month or two were allowed to elapse after its administration, clear-cut indications for *Pulsatilla* or other related medicines were sometimes thrown up. It is difficult to explain this other than by the supposition that *Carcinosin,* when indicated, has the power to disentanglce miasmatic influences.

CARCINOSIN

A clinical and pathogenetic study
By J. Hui Bon Hoa, M.D., D.F. Hom.

Gibson Miller liked to say that if he were confined to the use of one single remedy he would choose *Sepia*. I am sure that if this great homoeopath were alive today he would choose *Carcinosinum* which is the nosode, or should one rather say, the sarcode, of cancer. Following the work of Dr D. M. Foubister and Dr W. Lees Templeton of the Faculty of Homoeopathy of Great Britain, this remedy has come into current usage at the same level as *Sepia, Sulphur, Lycopodium, Phosphorus* and other constitutional remedies, surpassing them all in the number of times it is indicated.

The preparation used by Foubister and Templeton in clinical practice and in the elaboration of its pathogenesy is the original preparation of *Carcinosin*. Its origin is unknown. It was brought over from the United States and waa probably prepared from an epithelioma of the breast. A number of different specimens obtained from the operating theatre of the Royal London Homoeopathic Hospital are now available in potency. These *Carcinosins* were prepared by A. Nelson & Co. Six of them are now in current use. They are:

Carcinoma adeno stom— from an epithelioma of the stomach

Carcinoma adeno vesica—from an epithelioma of the bladder

Carcinoma intest. co.—from epitheliomata of the intestine and of the bladder

Carcinoma scir. mam.—from a scirrhus of the breast

Carcinoma squam. pulp.—from an epithelioma of the lung

The original *Carcinosin* of source unknown remains the one of choice because it alone has been the subject of considerable clinical and pathogenetic study. According to Foubister, the newer *Carcinosins* are extremely powerful and should be used with caution.

The time has now come to present to French-speaking homoeopaths a study of *Carcinosin* (modelled on the familiar style of Dr Duprat). The facts are drawn from the work of Dr D. M. Foubister who has described the general and mental characteristics of the remedy and drawn the drug picture in an article in the July 1958 number of *The British Homoeopathic Journal* which was translated into French by Dr E. Schepens of Brussels, and from that of Dr W. Lees Templeton who published a fine pathogenesy of this remedy in the April 1954 number of the same Journal.

I TABLE OF INDIVIDUAL CHARACTERISTICS

A TYPOLOGY

Physique

By reference to Foubister's list of related remedies and the classification of these remedies according to the biochemical constitutions of Vannier and Bernard we shall see that Carcinosin belongs equally to the carbonic (*Sulphur, Lycopodium*), phosphoric (*Nat. mur., Ara. alb., Phos,*) and sulphuric (of Bernard) (*Sulphur, Nat. sulph., Psorinum, Nat. mur.*) constitutions. None of the remedies described by Vannier as fluorique appear on Foubister's list.

Facies

Café-au-lait, pale complexion, with numerous moles and blue sclerotics (Foubister).

Psychology

Templeton's provings show up a sort of cerebral torpor, mental inertia which is aggravated by a feeling of cephalic constriction. The patient may even be apathetic and does not reply to questions. He is preoccupied, but annoyed by this. Brain work is a trial to him. Foubister has drawn attention to the beneficient action of *Carcinosin*, resembling that of *Medorrhinum,* in the treatment of mongols and sometimes other backward or mentally defective children. Dr J. H. Clarke wrote that *Carcinosin* was used in the treatment of psychotic patients with a tendency to suicide who had a cancerous heredity.

The following mental symptoms drawn from numerous clinical observations mainly from the work of Foubister are very important. Homoeopathic prescribing is based on this type of symptom, in addition to those obtained from provings.

Fundamental fear—prolonged fear, and prolonged unhappiness.

Anticipation. This takes the form of worry, sometimes amounting to anguish, as for example the late arrival of a child, husband, or wife, or the fear of young people that they may fail examinations. It is a frequent symptom of *Carcinosin* which has been of great value in my work. The list of remedies showing anxiety of anticipation thus becomes: *Arg. nit.,* Ars., Carbo. veg., CARC., *Gels.,* Lyc., Med., Plumb., Phos. ac., Sil., Thuja.

Attention to detail, exaggerated precision, fastidiousness, like ARS., *Nux v.,* Anac., Graph.

Obstinacy, like the *Tuberculins.*

Strong sense of rhythm, love of dancing; a useful confirmatory symptom of both *Sepia* and *Carcinosin.*

Sensitive to music which sometimes makes him weep. *Carc.,* Digitalis, GRAPH., *Kreos.,* Kali nit., NAT. C., Nat. sul., Nux v., *Thuja.* Note that *Nux* and *Carcinosin* are the only two remedies of the materia medica which both have fastidiousness and sensitivity to music. It is therefore useful to associate these two symptoms in our history taking, in the interests of rapid prescribing.

Like *Sepia* again, *Carcinosin* likes watching a thunderstorm.

Like *Phosphorus,* it is very sympathetic to others.

Like *Medorrhinum,* it is very sensitive to reprimand, a sycotic symptom, a pointed out by Dr Twentyman; found in the section of generalities, rubric "sycosis", of Kent's *Repertory.*

Finally, I have noticed that *Carcinosin* often has bizarre tics; one of my patients constantly tapped his brothers' skulls with his fingertips; another used to gently bite the tips of children's fingers, one after the other; he had not lost this habit at the age of 40. Sometimes *Carcinosin* tears at the skin round the nails. Dr Templeton points out that blinking of the eyes, another common form of tic, suggests *Carcinosin.* It has all sorts of grimaces.

All these symptoms are peculiar to *Carcinosin* and thus of great importance and we are indebted to Foubister for describing them.

B MODALITIES AND CHARACTERISTIC REACTIONS

Aggravation and *amelioration*

Aggravation or amelioration from heat or cold, or else the patient is sensitive to both heat and cold.

Very characteristic is the influence of the sea air, whether aggravation or amelioration, as in *Medorrhinum* and *Nat. mur. Medorrhinum* is characteristically better for sea air, very occasionally it has a seaside aggravation, whilst *Nat. mur.* has roughly 50% amelioration or aggravation. There may be aggravation on the Atlantic coast, amelioration on the Mediterranean coast, or vice versa. (The English equivalent, according to Foubister, is amelioration on the East coast and aggravation on the West coast, or vice versa.)

Worse for undressing (cough, skin), as in *Rumex*

Worse talking or laughing (cough), as in *Phos.*

Better after a short sleep

Causalities

A family history of cancer, diabetes, tuberculosis, pernicious anaemia, or a combination of these diseases more strongly represented than in an "average" family history (Foubister); hereditary syphilis (Cooper); a past history of whooping cough or other acute fevers at an early age.

Sensations

Beating, throbbing (Templeton)

Secretions

Acrid and thick

Desires and aversions (food)

Desire or aversion for salt, milk, eggs, fat, fruit.

Sometimes there is a desire in a child for one of these foods at one time, followed by aversion for the same food at another.

Alternation

Alternation of symptoms from one side of the body to the other as in *Lac caninum* and *Sepia*.

Periodicity

Afternoon, 1-6 p.m.

Concomitance

Numerous pigmented naevi, in particular, moles. Other remedies associated with pigmented naevi are: *Calc.*, Carb. v., Graph., Nitric ac., Petroleum, Phos. acid, PULS., Silicea, *Sulphur*, Sulph. ac., Tarentula, *Thuja*. Blue sclerotics, blinking of the eyes.

Sleep

Sleep disturbed. Difficulty in falling asleep, restless sleep; awakened by *shudders*; exciting dreams; over-active ideas (*Coffea*); lies awake most of the night; insomnia in general (Foubister).

Position during sleep

The child may sleep in the *genu-pectoral position* (position of Mohammedan prayer) as with *Medorrhinum*. Foubister's list of remedies associated with this position is as follows: *Carcinosin, Calc. phos., Lycopodium, Medorrhinum, Phos., Sepia, Tuberculinum.*

Dorsal position: with arms raised above the head (*Puls.*)

C GUIDING SYMPTOMS (W. L. Templeton)

Head

Throbbing headache. Pulsating, deep-seated, right-sided, suborbital headache (*Tub.*). Feeling of constriction of the brain.

Eyes

Twitching lids

Ear, nose and throat

Sensation as of a lump. Palatal pain, aggravated by hot drinks, ameliorated by cold; worse morning and evening (*Lach.*). (This localization to the palate is unusual and therefore of great importance, according to Templeton.)

Mouth

Tender gums, dental pain, ulceration

Chest

Cough; stomach cough (*Bry.*) provoked by tickling the substernal region. Aggravated by heat, in a warm room, or by cold air (*Rumex*); by laughing or talking (*Phos., Rumex*); from changing clothes (*Rumex*); from yawning (*Nat. sulph.*)

Cardiovascular system

Violent cardiac palpitation heard and felt by the patient (*Spigelia*). Feeling of constriction of the heart. Oppression of the chest, with the desire to take a deep breath (*Ignatia*).

Digestive system

Feeling of tightness, pain better for pressure or for bending, or for hot drinks (*Mag. phos.*). Constipation without desire (*Opium*). Stools hard and dry.

Back and limbs

Muscular *twitchings* in thighs, arms and back. Pain, weakness, fatigue and swelling of the thighs, better after a short sleep (marked symptoms). Pain in the legs, better for heat, or for gentle movement (*Puls.*), aggravated by *rapid* movement.

Skin

Acneiform eruption of the face. Rash between the shoulder-blades, worse for undressing (see cough).

II CLINICAL INDICATIONS

Mental retardation
Arthritis
Asthma
Headache
Mental confusion
Constipation
Neuro-vegetative dystonias
Ocular fatigue
Flatulence
Grimacing
Sexual impotence
Insomnia
Hepatic insufficiency
Masturbation
Migraine
Mongolism
Styes
Cardiac palpitation
Facial palsy

Intestinal parasitosis
Sacral pain
Sciatica
Tics
Cough
Ulceration of mucous membranes

On the subject of whether *Carcinosin* is indicated in cases of cancer Dr Foubister writes: "It must be noted that it is not without danger to give *Carcinosin* to cancer suspects." "It has often been used in the treatment of cancer. In an article published in the *Homoeopathic Recorder, Carcinosin* is claimed to relieve the pain of breast cancer; but there are no records of cases of cancer treated by *Carcinosin* alone, and it is doubtful whether it is of much value in the disease." Foubister's paper, however, deals with *Carcinosin* as a constitutional remedy and he says: "It seems that the further away you are from cancer, the more valuable it is as a constitutional remedy."

III ESSENTIAL FEATURES FOR THE PRESCRIPTION OF CARCINOSIN

Dr Foubister gives the following indications for the prescription of *Carcinosin:*

1. A family history of a tendency to cancer, diabetes, tuberculosis, pernicious anaemia, or a combination of these, a personal history of whooping cough or other severe acute infection at an early age.

2. Marked aggravation or improvement at the seaside.

3. Appetite: desire or aversion for salt, milk, eggs, fat, fruit.

4. Genu-pectoral position during sleep.

5. Associated remedies: the patient is partially covered by two or more of these remedies; or else apparently clearly indicated related remedies do not work, or have a very short action.

6. The appearance of the patient: moles, blue sclerotics or pale *café-au-lait* complexion.

One or more of the above conditions must be present.

IV RELATED AND COMPLEMENTARY REMEDIES

Tuberculins, Medorrhinum, Sepia, Syphilinum, Nat. mur., Calc. phos., Dys. co., Lycopodium, Phosphorus, Psorinum, Ars. alb., Ars. iod., Pulsatilla, Sulphur, Nat. sulph., Opium, Alumina, Staphysagria, Nux vomica, Dioscoria (Foubister). Associated bowel nosodes: *No growth, Cocci, Yeasts* (W. L. Templeton and J. Paterson).

Auto-isotherapy
Some patients who had responded to *Carcinosin* but whose improvement only lasted for a short time have derived benefit' from auto-isopathy. I give a single dose of *Pharyngeal Mucus* 30CH.

V POTENCIES

The following potencies are available from A. Nelson & Co., Ltd.:

C. adeno stom.	G	12	30	200	1M		
C. adeno vesica	6	12	30				
C. intest. co.	6	12	30				
C. scir. mam.	6	12	30	200			
C. squam. pulm.	6	12	30	200			
Old Carcinosin (on which this paper is based)			30	200	1M	10M	50M CM

VI CLINICAL CASES

CASE I (Dr Hui Bon Hoa)
This case was presented to the meeting of the *Société de Médecine Homoeopathique d'Aquitaine* on 11th March 1962.
Mme F., aged 78, sent by her doctor in September 1961 on account of jaundice which, in view of the patient's age, gave cause to suspect a neoplasm.

History of present condition
The illness began with mild fatigue which became rapidly worse, curtailing all physical activity, so that the patient, without being senile, found herself consigned to enforced rest, moving from chair to chair without being able to undertake any useful work whatever. Moreover, she developed angina of effort. It was then that she asked her doctor to obtain another opinion.

Past history revealed the following:
A severe attack of Spanish 'flu in 1917. She was expected to die, but recovered after a struggle.
Hypertension, 230/110, for which she was given Sarpagnan which upset her, followed by Anaprel which she tolerated better.
Her husband died of a growth of the colon. A grandmother also died of cancer.

On examination She was tired; she had an obvious *café-au-lait* complexion, but no jaundice. Liver and spleen were not enlarged. The stools were of normal colour, the urine normal and clear. Auscultation revealed extra systoles. Chest sounds normal. Reflexes normal. No lymphadenopathy.

Laboratory investigations
These showed a slight rise in the serum albumin and a right branch bundle block. Also diverticulous colon. Otherwise normal.

Individual characteristics
Typical *Carcinosin* appearance; *café-au-lait* complexion; enormous pigmented naevus of the forehead; multiple naevi; blue sclerotics. Feels the heat.
Meticulous and fastidious.
Anticipatory anxiety.

Conclusion
An asthenic patient, whose typical *Carcinosin.* skin had given rise to an impression of icterus. Precancerous condition. A typical *Carcinosin* from both the morphological and psychological points of view.
Treatment: Carcinosin 200 one dose.
Results: Marked improvement from the 7th day of treatment. The asthenia and precordial pain disappeared and the patient resumed her normal activity. There was no aggravation.
On 23rd February 1962 this patient was still well. Her appearance was unchanged. B.P. 190/100. No medicine.

CASE II
Mme B., aged 42, governess, had suffered for eight days from pain in the right buttock, of moderate severity, which prevented her from sleeping.

Modalities
Worse for stumbling
Worse for sitting in one position for long
Worse lying down
Better standing

On examination
Lasegue's sign
A fibrous band, two centimetres long, and as thick as a pencil, was present on the right border of the sacrum, and gave rise to pain which radiated to the anal fold.
Blue sclerotics
A few moles

Carcinosin 200 CH, 1 dose.
The pain had distinctly improved the day after the administration of the remedy, and had completely disappeared by the following day. At the same time, the patient experienced a general sense of well-being, great euphoria, and increased vitality. There was no aggravation.
Other symptoms were as follows:
Sensitive to heat
Desire for sweets
Desire for strongly seasoned food
Sensitive to music
Sensitive to noise
Sensitive to reprimand
Cutaneous hyperaesthesia
Anticipatory anxiety

Past history
Childish ailments
Serious croup at 5
Chronic leucorrhoea as a small girl
Her father and two of his brothers died of cancer
No tuberculosis in the family

CASE III
Mme B., aged 38, no profession, suffered from asthma. The attacks came every evening at bedtime, never during

the day. They were not very severe, but wheezing forced her to get up. They responded to theophyline suppositories. Her asthma was ameliorated by liver extracts, aggravated after such food as fried food, port and shellfish.

Past history
Infantile asthma till puberty (at 12 years) and again from age 30 until the present.
Whooping cough. Possibly initiated the disease.
Heredity. Maternal grandmother died of cancer.
Collateral relatives. A first cousin and a nephew asthmatic.

On examination

Respiration completely normal (attacks only occur at night), but considerable abdominal meteorism. Liver not enlarged or tender. The lower limbs were very thin by comparison with the average corpulence of her body. Multiple *large moles.*

No other findings. Cholesterol 1.30 g.

She had had extensive homoeopathic treatment in another town. One frequently meets with a case such as this, where *Pertussin, Carbo. veg., Nux vomica* and *Streptococcin* and other remedies have been prescribed with good results.

The following mental and general symptoms were also present:
Worse for heat
Better in open air
Worse for wind
Worse at new moon
Not affected by storms or the seaside
Hunger easily satisfied

Desire for sugar
Desire for hot drinks
Dislikes fat
Irregular, restless sleep
Nervous and distrait, easily gets angry when contradicted
Afraid of having cancer like her mother
Tidy, but not excessively so
Not particularly sensitive to music
Many large moles
All these symptoms were very definite.

Lycopodium 30 CH which was apparently indicated, gave no result, so for the following reasons:

1 The apparently well indicated related remedy did not work,
2 Family history of cancer,
3 Presence of large moles,
4 *Lycopodium* does not cover fear of illness and is complementary to *Carcinosin,* a single dose of *Carcinosin* 200 was given and the patient recovered in 9 days (including flatulence and leucorrhoea which she had not mentioned) without aggravation.

CASE IV

Mme J., aged 52, no profession, suffered from insomnia. She had slept badly since the age of 15 and this was getting worse. She could spend a whole night without shutting her eyes (Dr Templeton's pathogenesy). Weeps while giving the history (*Kali. c., Med., PULS.,* SEP.).

Past history
Hysterectomy for fibroids three years ago. Post-operative phlebitis with two emboli. Pentothal anaeathesia.
Grandfather died of cancer

One uncle had tuberculosis
One aunt had tuberculosis
One cousin had tuberculosis

Physical examination
Nothing was noteworthy, except perhaps for a chronic reddening of the conjunctivae.
The general and mental symptoms were as follows:
Worse from heat, or in a warm room
Better in the open air
Must have fresh air
Aversion from fat
Aggravation from milk
Good character
Excessively timid
Weeps easily
Weeps whilst giving her history to the doctor
Very sensitive and emotional
Would like consolation, but says there is no one to console her
Declares that ordinary drugs poison her
One enormous mole on her back (*Puls*. very frequently has this sign also)
All very definite symptoms.

Pulsatilla 7 CH, 9 CH, 30 CH was given on three successive days, without effect.
So for the following reasons:
1 The apparently indicated remedy had no effect,
2 Family history of cancer and tuberculosis,
3 Presence of a large mole on the back,
4 *Pulsatilla* is complementary to *Carcinosin*, a single dose of *Carcinosin* 200 was given which cured the patient without aggravation.

CASE V

Mme M., aged 26, no profession, consulted me for chronic discoloration of the skin. The anamnesis revealed that she suffered from migraine, constipation and insomnia.

Past history
Typhoid $2\frac{1}{2}$ years; purulent peritonitis at 8 years; diphtheria; measles; chicken pox.

Family history
Her father died of uraemia; her grandmother died of carcinoma of the rectum.

There was no tuberculosis in the family.

The general and mental symptoms were as follows:
Very chilly
Stifled in a hot room
Worse before and during a storm
Desire for eggs
Desires spiced food
Sleeps on her stomach
Highly strung; starts at a sudden noise
Better for physical exercise
Many moles

Physical examination
The conjunctivae and skin were discoloured yellow. The liver was of normal size and not tender to palpation. The spleen was not felt. There was no abdominal meteorism or other abnormality on clinical examination.

Carcinosin 200 CH 1 dose was given.

The patient was very upset immediately after *Carcinosin* was administered, and I took advantage of this reaction to give an acupuncture treatment as follows.

T.R.10., T.R.3., M.C.6., V.60., E.45., V.13.

Equilibrium was at once restored.

From the second day after treatment had started, the icterus began to fade and disappeared completely together with the insomnia, constipation and migraine.

The interesting thing about this case was the canalization of the reaction by acupuncture. In connection with this, Dr. Foubister has often observed a febrile reaction on the tenth day after administration of *Carcinosin*—a reaction which he points out can best be understood if it is agreed with Macdonagh and Rudolf Steiner that there are two fundamental disease processes: inflammation and tumour formation. This febrile reaction or a past history of severe early infectious disease can be considered as a reaction against hereditary cancerous tendencies.

APPENDIX

SCIRRHINUM

Burnett was one of the first homoeopaths to use *Carcinosin* to any extent and he was followed by Clarke. Apart from *Carcinosin* one of his favourite remedies was *Scirrhinum,* or *Durum,* prepared from a scirrhus carcinoma. Its key-note was *"a violent feeling of hollowness"* at the umbilicus. Burnett claimed to have cured numerous cases of tumour of the breast with this remedy. He also cured a gross indurated cervical adenopathy, cases of haemorrhage, and varices of the lower limbs. One patient expelled a considerable number of *threadworms* after the administration of *Scirrhinum.* In obstinate cases of this kind, where *Cina* or *Teucrium* had no effect, Clarke, whose notes provide this information, obtained good results with *Scirrhinum* 200. Its time of aggravation is from 5-6 p.m., and irregularly throughout the night.

CARCINOMA

Kent comments in *Lesser Writings* p. 411:

"*Carcinoma* relieves pain that is sharp, burning or tearing. With this remedy (a nosode) patients remained comfortable for many years, even though cure was impossible and the cancer continued to develop. The growth of the tumour was delayed, and the suffering, which usually goes with this condition, was avoided.

"The preparation of *Carcinoma* which I have used for come years was taken from a cancer of the breast. The patient had a permanent, clear, colorless watery discharge. A small quantity of this liquid was potentized and has been used with good effect in many cases of advanced epithelioma."

MICROCOCCINUM AND OSCILLOCOCCIN

Two French remedies similar to *Carcinosin*.

Micrococcinum was prepared from *Micrococcus neoformans,* which was found in a malignant tumour by Doyen in 1901, and which he held to be the cause of cancer. *Micrococcinum* has been used by Léon Vannier since 1919 as a "specific desensitizer of the cancerinic state".

Oscillococcin was prepared from the oscillococcus described by a homoeopathic physician, Dr Roy, in 1925. It also was soon used by Léon Vannier. Vannier himself described the results of his experiment: "In the cancerinic state, *Micrococcinum* and *Oscillococcin* are far from giving the same results as the potentised tuberculins give in the tuberculinique state. Nevertheless, in certain cancerinic states a change can take place under their influence. In particular, loss of weight can be arrested almost immediately, but this continuity of action cannot be compared with that of the *Tuberculins*" (Les Canceriniques). On the other hand, Vannier was much more impressed by *auto-isotherapy* with blood.

Oscillococcin is better known for its action against influenza. There are no key-notes: it seems to work as a pathological remedy for influenza (Chavanon).

BIBLIOGRAPHY

Bernard, H., *Traité de médecine homéopathique.*

Boericke, E., *Pocket manual of homoeopathic materia medica,* 9th edition.

Clarke, J., *A dictionary of practical materia medica,* 3rd edition, 3 vol.

Foubister, D.M., *Brit. Hom. Journal,* "The Carcinosin Drug Picture", 47, 201, July 1958.

Kent, J.T., *New remedies, Clinical cases, Lesser writings.*

Kent, J.T., *Aphorisms and Precepts,* 1st Indian edition.

Templeton, W.L., *The British Homoeopathic Journal,* April 1954.

Vannier, L., *La Typologie et ses applications thérapeutiques, 1re partie: Generalities et Constitutions.*

Vannier, L., *Les Canceriniques et leur traitement homeopathique.*